Heal Your Foot Wound Fast

Dr. Donald Pelto

TABLE OF CONTENTS

INTRODUCTION

Learning how to heal foot wounds quickly is one of the most important things you should know if you have a wound or if you care for someone with a foot wound. Wounds can be a result of many disease processes such as neuropathy, diabetes and injury.

Finding reliable information about caring for foot wounds can be very confusing. There may be loads of information available at the click of a mouse, but the amount of online resources can overwhelm you very quickly. Some of the information online may be part of a commercial sales pitch, and even independent information is not always reliable.

The Heal Your Foot Wound Fast book, however, is based on sound medical facts from a podiatrist who specializes in diabetic foot care.

What is the best way to heal a foot wound?

And how can you heal a foot wound quickly?

The Heal Your Foot Wound Fast book will answer those questions simply and directly.

As a podiatrist with specific experience treating foot wounds, I will walk you through very specific steps to healing foot wounds quickly. You will also learn about ways to keep your feet healthy so that you have fewer problems and thereby prevent foot wounds to begin with.

Why 'Quick' Matters

It may seem like common sense to want to heal a foot wound quickly— and it is.

But why? The longer a foot wound exists, the greater your risk for very serious complications. Speed in treating and healing a foot wound can stop other problems from developing.

The longer a wound on the foot is open, the greater your risk of developing an infection or even amputation. In fact, foot wounds in people with diabetes are the leading cause of amputation. Amputation may seem like a far-off possibility—but it may not be far away if you are walking on a foot wound and not treating it properly to help it heal quickly—especially if you are not seeing a podiatrist or other physician.

Take charge of preventing these extreme problems!

How To Use The Heal Your Foot Wound Fast Book

This book explains nine steps for healing wounds quickly—perhaps more quickly than you have been able to heal foot wounds in the past.

Many patients and their caregivers tell me that they have heard this advice before, and you may have heard some or all of this before, too. **It is important to understand and follow all of the steps to help heal foot wounds quickly and prevent infection, which can lead to amputation.**

Each of the nine steps is important, and they are all related to one another. You will be integrating the steps into things that you are already doing as part of your own care.

Healing foot wounds is not necessarily a simple process; you need to understand the steps and follow all of them. This guide is *not* a replacement for having a podiatrist, a vascular surgeon or an endocrinologist involved in the wound care team.

If you are living in a country where you do not have podiatrists or access to a wound care team, we will give you and your care provider a solid treatment plan to help prevent amputation.

Each section of the guide will address one of the nine steps in detail. Some of the steps deal with factors surrounding your general diabetes care and/or foot care. Remember, all are important!

1. **Get and keep control of your nutrition and blood sugar**

   The truth is that many people who have foot wounds also have diabetes. Nutrition is one of many important factors that affect diabetes. In addition to affecting blood sugar levels and weight, nutrition also plays a role in helping foot wounds heal.

2. **Evaluate blood flow and swelling**

   Poor blood flow and swelling can slow down the healing foot wounds. Learn how to evaluate your blood flow, control swelling and work with a vascular specialist (a doctor who is an expert in blood circulation.)

3. **Understand and perform a wound evaluation**

   The skin around the wound is important. What does it look and feel like? Is it red, hard, calloused, black or darkened, or bruised? These are important clues about infection, bruises and other issues.

4. **Assess your foot construction and function**

   Bones, tendons and muscles are all involved in the wound healing process. How are your feet constructed and functioning? Are there any tight tendons that are contributing to added pressure on your foot? Are there areas where bones protrude? Do you have a flat or a very high foot? Is your arch collapsed?

5. **Evaluate your nerves**

   How is the feeling in your foot? Do you have a condition called neuropathy (a lack of feeling in your feet or numbness in your feet)? How do you determine your feeling? All are important factors to healing foot wounds quickly.

6. Examine and evaluate your wound and treatments used

Look at the type of wound you have. Is it granular, red and beefy, or white?

And evaluate the types of treatments you have been using. Have you had the actual tissue around the wound removed? Have you been having different types of products or medications placed in the wound to remove all the unhealthy tissue?

7. Understand wound care dressings

Examine the actual wound, the type of dressings you are using, and how often you are changing them. Options that can help your wound heal more quickly are abundant. Some of them include wet-to-moist, betadine, gels, foams, alginates, hydrocolloids and new types of skin grafts and artificial skin substitutes.

8. Take the pressure off your wound

Every wound needs to be "off-loaded"; that is, you have to take the pressure off of it for the wound to heal. What type of off-loading are you doing, and is it correct for the type and location of your wound? If a shoe is causing the problem, do you have an improper shoe that is not allowing your foot wound to heal? If so, learn where to find the proper shoes and if you may qualify for diabetic shoes.

9. Prevent foot wounds from occurring again

Learn who should be on your diabetic care team once your wound has healed so that you can prevent the wound from recurring. What are some of the other complications of diabetes that can affect your wound healing, and how can you help protect yourself from those complications?

Caution! Before you dive into the steps...

The details presented in this e-book should never be a substitute for seeing your own doctor. You should be seeing a podiatrist, a vascular specialist or a wound care center in your area, if that is possible. Listen to your wound care clinician and try to do all that you can for yourself to help your foot wound heal fast.

Heal Your Foot Wound Fast is for educational purposes only. It is not a substitute for treatment!

The next chapter is a summary of the 9 Steps. This will outline each step and give you a link to each of the steps so you can listen, read or watch the content.

To your health,

Dr. Donald Pelto

FOOT WOUND SCORECARD®

Prior to learning about the wound healing steps, here is a Wound Healing Scorecard® for you to evaluate your current situation. It would be good to go over this scorecard to see where you are; and then after, periodically review where you are at in terms of your wound recovery and knowledge.

Foot Wound Scorecard®

		1 – 2 – 3	4 – 5 – 6	7 – 8 – 9	10 – 11 – 12	Score
1	Blood Sugar and Nutrition	My blood sugar is under control daily, my Hemoglobin A1C is under 7 and has always been that way. I am eating well and focusing on protein.	My blood sugar is okay and my Hemoglobin A1C is around 7 but in the past it has been much higher. I try to eat well with protein.	My blood sugar is very high and my A1C is between 7-10. I am frustrated and discouraged. As well I don't eat regularly and have difficulty with diet.	I can't ever get my blood sugar under control even with my doctor's help and medications. I do not eat well because good food is expensive.	
2	Blood Flow and Swelling	I have excellent blood flow. I have had circulation studies and my blood flow is normal. I have no swelling.	I have good blood flow but because of my swelling it is difficult to feel my pulses. I have had circulation exam and my blood flow is okay.	I have either one or both of my pulses that can not be felt. I have not had a blood flow study and not seen a doctor. I have bad swelling also.	I have very bad circulation problems. My toes are discolored and cold all the time. I have not seen a doctor because I am scared what I will find.	
3	Skin and Wound Evaluation	My wound is a red color and is scabbing over and healing in well.	My wound is healthy red color but it is very deep. The skin around the wound looks normal and no infection.	My wound is not healthy in color and the skin around it is swollen and discolored.	My wound is very deep and going down to bone. There is redness (cellulitis) around my foot.	
4	Bone and Pressure Evaluation	I know where I have high areas of pressure that are at risk for an ulceration. I have special shoes to help reduce pressure on foot.	I know where I have high pressure areas on my foot but don't want to wear any special shoes or boots because of the way that they look.	I don't know what the cause of my wound and don't know how pressure contributes my foot wound but I want to learn more.	I am not interested in knowing how pressure contributes to my wound and think my doctor should do everything.	
5	Nerves and Feeling Evaluation	I do not have any neuropathy and have no lack of feeling in my feet. I get tested every year.	I have the beginnings of neuropathy and I get tested yearly to see how much feeling I have in my feet.	I have painful neuropathy and I am being tested and treated by my doctor.	I can't feel my feet but I have never seen a doctor to be tested for neuropathy. I stop on ground so I can feel something while walking.	
6	Wound Debridement and Surgery	My wound was debrided once and then it got better and I get frequent callus care to prevent recurrence.	My wound is slow to heal but I get frequent wound care (every 1-2 weeks) and I don't need surgery.	I see a doctor regularly for wound debridement and since my wound won't heal I will need surgery.	I don't see a doctor but do my own debriding of my wound with a razor blade to cut off the dead skin.	
7	Wound Dressings and Grafts	I only needed a little triple antibiotic ointment and my wound healed quickly.	I use some advanced wound dressings on my wound that I get from my doctor and my wound is improving.	I have had a skin graft to help my wound healing and it is healthy and doing well.	I don't know what to put on my wound to help it heal. I don't have a doctor and am scared.	
8	Shoes and Off-Loading	I wear diabetic shoes and I like wearing them and switch my shoe inserts every 3 months.	I have a special shoe or boot to off-load the pressure on my foot. I wear this all the time even at home.	I have a special boot or shoe to wear but I don't wear it at home and only sometimes when out of the house.	Diabetic shoes are ugly and my doctor wants me to wear a special for my wound but I don't want to.	
	Scorecard	➡ ➡ ➡ ➡	➡ ➡ ➡ ➡	➡ ➡ ➡ ➡	➡ ➡ ➡ ➡	

Scoring System

0-24 - You probably don't have a problem foot wound at this time or your problem is very mild. Minimal treatment is needed but daily foot checks are important to avoid any further problems.

25-48 - You have mild wound that is being well taken care of. You understand the treatments that are needed to heal your foot wound and have the appropriate shoe gear that is needed. Frequent visits to the doctor are needed to help monitor your foot wound until it is healed.

49-72 - You have severe symptoms in your overall health that is making it harder to heal your foot wound. You should be following up with your doctor or podiatrist on a regular basis to make sure there are no further problems or infections. You are at high risk for having bone infection or even amputation and close care is needed. It is good for you to read the information in this publication to understand more about the risks and the proper treatments for healing your foot wound.

73-96 - You have a severe foot wound and need help urgently. You may have other conditions like poor feeling (neuropathy) or poor blood flow (peripheral arterial disease) or even an infection. All of these make you at high risk for further problems. Even if your wound heals over time you need frequent podiatry care to prevent further issues.

9 STEP SUMMARIES

This is a quick summary of the 9 steps of how to heal your wounds fast. For more details, please read all of the full sections that are linked to each number because they provide a lot of important information for you to know. If you are diabetic and/or neuropathic, please read the steps so that you know how to help heal your wound. If you don't currently have a wound or have never had one, please read the steps anyway so that you know how to prevent wounds.

STEP 1: **Blood Sugar and Nutrition:** Many factors affect the healing of your foot wound, including your general health, nutrition, and keeping your diabetes under control. Here are some tips on how to have good health and nutrition when you're diabetic:

You should be checking your blood sugar several times a day. Levels may be between 89-120.

Know your hemoglobin A1C test value. This is a long-term measure of how well you're doing with your blood sugar. It should be no higher than 7.

Don't just depend on medications to keep your diabetes "under control".

If you need to lose weight, you can do this by eating less, eating healthy, or increasing exercise activity.

Stop eating when you feel full. Eat slowly so you notice this.

Drink lots of water

Don't eat in front of the TV or other distractions

Take control of your health and nutrition because staying healthy helps wound healing

Consider using intermittent fasting as a way to reduce weight and control blood sugars

STEP 2: Blood Flow and Swelling: We need good blood flow to keep us healthy. Here are some quick tips on things you should check for to make sure you have good blood flow:

Pulses in your feet (see the detailed Step 2 on how to do this)

Make sure there is no swelling in your legs or feet, which can prevent or stop your wound from healing

Don't be afraid to ask your doctor if you need to see a vascular surgeon

STEP 3: Skin and Wound Evaluation: Skin can tell us a lot about how healthy we are - so take a careful look at your wound and the area around it. Here are some quick tips on what to look for and do:

Check your feet or have someone else check them regularly. Be creative and find a way to do this.

Use lotion or cream on dry skin, but NOT between the toes.

Calluses are bad because they create pressure and pressure = possible future wound

Look at wound color, edges, drainage, and surrounding skin. Notice any bad odor.

Special occasion shoes that hurt even when worn only for a couple hours can cause blisters and blisters = possible future wound

No excuses...check your feet and wound daily!

STEP 4: Bone and Pressure Evaluation: Bony prominences on our feet can be pressure areas when we walk and pressure areas = possible future wound. Here are some things that cause wounds:

Bony prominences! This includes bunions and hammertoes.

Calluses and corns are areas of bony prominences, and these are bad.

A tight heel cord forces pressure elsewhere, so stretch it out!

A Charcot foot is a red, hot, swollen, rocker-bottom foot that basically has a lot of small fractures within it. Go see your doctor if you feel like this describes your foot type.

Make sure you're always asking, "What's causing my wound?"

STEP 5: Nerves and Sensation: Pain is a gift because it's our body's warning signal that something is wrong. A lack of pain sensation, also called neuropathy, is dangerous for diabetics. Here are some things to know about your pain sensations:

Being able to experience pain is a good thing

High blood sugar can make nerves swell and delay their warning signals to us

There is no guaranteed cure for injured nerves

Ask your doctor if you need a test for the nerves in your feet

If you're diabetic AND neuropathic, walking a lot can create calluses and pressure areas (which = possible future wounds).

STEP 6: Wound Debridement and Surgery: Any callus and bad tissue covering your wound needs to be 'debrided' or removed because this can prevent your wound from healing. Don't remove any skin or tissue yourself! Visit a doctor so this can be done in a clean environment with the right tools.

Calluses and corns need to be trimmed by a professional because they can cause wounds

The ideal wound is one where the tissue is red and healthy looking

Bleeding is not bad. It means your body has the ability to heal your wound.

Your doctor is happy when your wound bleeds. You should be too.

Wound cultures can trick us because our skin normally has bacteria on it

Bone infection is bad and may mean the bone needs to be removed

Wounds present for many years may need a biopsy because they can turn into a type of cancer.

STEP 7: Wound Dressings and Grafts: Wounds should really be covered with dressings for protection and padding. There are a lot of different dressings out there, so here are some tips on which dressing may be right for you:

A thin clear film on your wound is biofilm. It's like soap scum that sits on top of your wound. It prevents your wound from healing and needs to be removed.

A wound with A LOT of drainage needs a seaweed (or alginate) dressing to absorb drainage and bacteria.

Deep AND draining wounds need a foam dressing.

Black or dry wounds need a hydrogel to keep it moist.

Wounds with healthy, red tissue can use a hydrogel too.

Yellow, fibrous wounds are challenging. This tissue needs to turn red and healthy.

Infected wounds benefit from iodine or a silver dressing (it doesn't actually look like jewelry).

Make sure your dressing is getting changed regularly.

If your wound hasn't been healing quickly, ask your doctor about 'skin substitutes.'

The most important thing to remember is that bad tissue needs to be removed!

STEP 8: Shoes and Off-Loading: You really shouldn't be walking a lot if you have a foot wound. Track how much you're walking, even at home. You'd be surprised to learn how much you walk around your house. Here are some tips about how to take pressure off your wound:

Ask your doctor about special shoes/devices to help off-load your foot. These include a roll-about, wheelchair, total contact cast, removable cast walker, half-shoe, and surgical shoe. All of them work to get pressure OFF of the bottom of your foot.

Have your foot measured. You're probably wearing the wrong size shoe, and this is bad.

Shoes are VERY important. Make sure you're wearing the right shoe AND size!

STEP 9: Preventing Recurrence and Other Complications: So you've managed to heal your foot wound fast. What happens now? Well, you want to prevent another wound because once you've had a wound, you're more likely to get another one. Here are some tips on what to do now:

Continue to check your feet daily!

Get a diabetic foot exam. How often this happens will depend on your blood flow, foot type, and sensation. You might have to get an exam anywhere from every 2 months to once a year.

Podiatrists don't just trim your nails and calluses so your feet will look good. They do this to help prevent wounds.

Get diabetic shoes. They help prevent wounds.

Wear your diabetic shoes at home. At least wear SOMETHING that will protect your feet if you bump into things.

Your healthcare team is made up of people who work together to help you stay healthy. It can include a blood flow doctor, infectious disease doctor, skin doctor, physical therapist, pedorthist (shoe specialist), cast technician, visiting home nurse, dietician, endocrinologist, primary care or family doctor, kidney doctor, eye doctor, and/or brain doctor.

Thank you for reviewing all of these steps on how to heal your foot wound fast and again, please read the detailed steps for ALL of the info. I hope you have learned a lot!

STEP 1: BLOOD SUGAR AND NUTRITION

What Blood Sugar and Nutrition Means for Healing Wounds Fast

Many factors affect healing a foot wound, including your general health, nutrition and keeping your diabetes under control.

Your nutrition actually can have a big impact on general health, diabetes and healing foot wounds.

Keeping Diabetes Under Control

First, you need to be sure you know what "out of control" means for your diabetes. "Control" is measured in different ways.

If you have diabetes, you are probably checking your blood sugar levels throughout the day. If you have a foot wound, you might be checking your blood sugar levels hourly. Blood sugar levels may vary throughout the day, depending on when you have last eaten. Levels may range between 89 and 120.

Another test to measure control of your diabetes is the hemoglobin A1C test. The hemoglobin A1C test can explain how well your blood sugar is over the last three months. It is a very effective exam. In this test, your doctor or staff draws your blood. The number you want from this test is about a 7.

What if the hemoglobin A1C test shows and 8, 9 or10? That would reflect problem of having a high amount of blood sugar in your system over time. The higher level of sugar in your blood actually slows down your body's ability to heal wounds.

When you test your blood sugar levels throughout the day, a spike from a usual 80 or 90 to 300 could signal a foot wound or an infection in a foot wound. This is because any additional stress on your body—like a wound or an infection—can cause your blood sugar to rise.

Keeping a close eye on blood sugar levels not only helps control diabetes on a daily basis but also helps identify a wound or infection and can help you assess how your body is healing a wound.

Balancing Nutrition, Medication and Weight Loss

Balancing nutrition, medication and weight loss is a challenge for everyone. It can become a bigger challenge if you have a foot wound.

Most people with diabetes are trying to control their nutrition for their diabetes, and many are also taking medicine (pills or insulin). Many are also trying to lose weight. That is a lot to balance, but doing so can keep you healthy and help your body heal wounds quickly.

To lose weight you need to eat less, eat differently and/or increase the amount of your daily activity.

But, if you have a foot wound you cannot do anything. You cannot run or walk. It is hard to get around, and it is hard to do those types of physical activities. It can become very stressful on people because controlling weight can be so challenging if you cannot work out.

Here are three tips on how you can control your weight if you have diabetes.

1. Stop eating when you are still hungry. Many of us are programmed from our childhood to do the opposite when our parents said, "I want you to clean your plate."

   But it is important to stop eating when you are still hungry. There are two ways of doing that. One: put less food on your plate. Two: use a smaller plate that will hold less food.

2. Consider intermittent fasting. This is a method of control of diabetes and weight loss that uses longer periods of alternate day fasting for health reasons. If you consider starting intermittent fasting and you have diabetes, discuss this with your doctor or endocrinologist. There are many resources online to learn about intermittent fasting that are beyond the scope of this book.

3. Drink a lot of water—not a lot of coffee, tea, diet soda or anything caffeinated.

Simply carrying water throughout your day and drinking it is going to help you control your weight and increase hydration for your overall health.

I use the reusable plastic bottles you would clip onto a bicycle. I try to drink two of them in the morning, two after lunch and another two before bed. I leave them out and close at hand so that it becomes a habit to drink them every day.

Wherever you go carry water so that you have it handy to drink

Types of Foods and Nutrients—and how They Impact Foot Wounds

The types of foods you eat when you have a diabetic foot wound can affect the wound and your body's ability to heal it quickly.

When you have a chronic wound or when you have a wound on your foot, you need to assess your nutrition. Many patients need to work with a nutritionist to assess and revamp their nutrition; this can play a major role in helping you heal a wound quickly and prevent major problems.

All foot wounds can put a high demand for nutrients in your body. Wounds that are infected increase the demand for nutrients in your body because the infection damages tissue and adds strain on your body and overall health. When you have a foot wound, your body loses a lot of elements or nutrients that are carried throughout your body. You need to be sure you are eating enough of the right nutrients to keep up with your body's demand for them while your foot wound is healing.

Protein

If you have a wound that is draining a lot and you are changing the dressing a couple of times a day, you are losing a lot of the different elements that your body needs to keep it healthy and help fight infection.

In particular, your body loses a lot of protein through the wound. Your body needs protein to heal. One type of blood test checks the albumin level in your blood and can be a good indicator of your overall health. We find that people who are in the hospital after having foot surgery and/or have a wound that is slow to heal need to work with a nutritionist to get the right balance of nutrients and protein to help their bodies heal.

Beef, fish, poultry, pork, peanut butter and beans are high in protein, and you should eat two to three servings of these foods each day. Sometimes drinking protein shakes or a meal replacement drink high in protein can help your body heal wounds.

You must have enough protein!

Blood Sugar & Nutrients

As always, you need to monitor your blood sugar and continue to eat the right types of foods to keep your diabetes under control when you are healing a foot wound.

Many other nutrients are very important for healing foot wounds. They include vitamin A, vitamin C and zinc among others. You may need to talk with your dietician or even with your endocrinologist to get the right nutritional balance while a foot wound heals.

Remember: controlling your diabetes and your weight and eating the right amounts of nutrients will help you heal foot wounds quickly. If your wound is healing slowly or not improving, your nutrition may be a reason.

STEP 2: BLOOD FLOW AND SWELLING

What Blood Flow Means for Healing Wounds Fast

Blood flow is what keeps our bodies healthy. If you have a wound on your foot (or anywhere on your body), blood is what brings nutrients to the area to help heal it and wash away any infection.

How does the foot get blood to it? The foot has two main arteries that bring it blood. Here are also veins that bring blood back to the heart. If an artery is blocked, this can slow blood flow to the foot, making it hard for a wound to heal. You may hear doctors talk about "pulses," which really means blood flow. How good is your blood flow? Common questions people ask are "Will I lose my foot?" or "Will my foot turn black?" A person with good pulses or blood flow should not lose their entire foot due to a small toe with gangrene (death of tissue).

Clogged arteries and thus poor pulses to the foot are 20 times more likely to cause a loss of a foot if you have diabetes. You also have a 60 times greater chance of developing gangrene. Most amputations occur in people with diabetes, but not in people with diabetes AND good pulses. So you may ask, "How do I know if I have good pulses?" This is something you can check yourself, right now.

We have two main pulses in our feet that can be easily felt, or palpated as doctors like to say. The first pulse can be felt by putting two fingers on the top of your foot between your first and second toes, then moving your fingers backwards towards your ankle about 2-3 inches. This pulse is called dorsalis pedis. If you can feel this, then you have good blood flow to the top of your foot. The second pulse can be found on the inside of the ankle, just behind the ankle bone. This pulse is called the posterior tibial pulse. If you can feel this pulse, then you have good blood flow to the bottom of your foot.

When Pulses Can't Be Felt

There are a couple of common tests that can be done to evaluate blood flow in your legs. The most common test is called an Ankle-Brachial Index, or what doctors like to call "ABI." An ABI is done by placing blood pressure cuffs (the same one that gets put on your arm when you go for checkups) on your legs. These are placed on your thigh, right above your knee, right below your knee, and at the toe. These are then inflated to measure your blood pressure and the values are compared to the blood pressure in your arm. If the values are the same, good news! If any of the values in your legs are lower than the arm, then there may be some clogging in your arteries. This can help diagnose something called PAD, or peripheral arterial disease (meaning poor blood flow).

What is PAD? What does PAD mean to you? How does this happen? PAD, happens when fat or "plaque" gets stuck in the arteries. If these block the flow to your heart, this will increase your chance for a heart attack because your heart isn't getting enough blood and has to work a lot harder than normal. If your blood flow is decreased in the arteries in your neck, then blood flow to your brain is decreased. This can lead to a stroke. Clogging of the arteries in your feet work the same way. Without good blood flow to your feet, this could cause a wound to develop, a wound to heal slowly, or even gangrene.

Symptoms of PAD

There is a questionnaire that we and other doctors use to screen for PAD. If you can respond 'yes' to any of the following questions, then you may want to ask your doctor if you need an ABI. First, do you have any calf, thigh, hip, or buttock discomfort? Do you experience any aching, fatigue, tingling, or cramping type pain when you walk? Does this go away when you rest, which helps you walk again? Second, do you experience any pain in your lower legs or feet when you're resting at home just sitting around or laying in bed? Third, do you have any pain in your toes, feet, legs, or thighs that disturbs your sleep? Or do your toes look pale or blue? Other questions to answer: Has a doctor ever told you that you have diminished pulses? Have you ever had a foot wound before? Have you had a foot infection before? Have you ever had black discoloration to your toes or feet?

Again, if you can answer yes to any of these questions, it would be good to consider getting an Ankle-Brachial Index study, or ABI.

Blood Vessel Studies

There are more advanced tests that can also be done, such as an MRA, or magnetic resonance angiography. Yes, it's like an MRI for your blood vessels. This is a way to look at the arteries themselves and to see exactly where any clogging is. Sometimes a clog can be bad enough that the doctor will use a device to open up the artery or remove the plaque.

Why is blood flow so important? Some people have infected wounds that need to be treated with antibiotics medications. For example, if you take an antibiotic for an infection, the antibiotic cannot reach your wound if there is no blood to carry it there.

The first goal in addressing the infected wound is to make sure there is good blood flow to bring the antibiotic to the area. The second goal is to make sure you're on the right antibiotic for your particular wound. For some people, they have to have antibiotics through their veins because their wounds are too deep or have too bad of an infection. People with really bad blood flow may even need antibiotic beads, which are placed directly into the wound. This allows you to get a more concentrated amount of antibiotic without depending on blood flow.

A Breakdown of Swelling

What about swelling? What does swelling mean for healing wounds fast? This also goes back to blood flow and those veins we discussed earlier. Legs can swell if your heart can't pump the blood so it instead goes backwards, because the veins can't bring the blood back to your heart. Swelling can slow the movement of blood flow, which slows wound healing.

The wound itself can also be a way for your body to get rid of all the extra fluid so you may see a lot of drainage. When this fluid drains, you can lose the nutrients and protein needed to heal wounds fast. Again, I stress the importance of good nutrition.

So how can you control any swelling? Swelling can be controlled through a few ways, including medications that help get rid of the extra fluid. These are called 'water pills,' which a lot of people don't like to take if they're far from home because they do cause frequent bathroom trips.

Other ways to control swelling include compression wraps or dressings. Profore is a common dressing that starts at the foot and goes up the leg.

Things to remember: If your wound isn't healing, and your blood sugar and nutrition are "under control," then consider how good your blood flow is or how much swelling you have in your legs and feet.

STEP 3: SKIN AND WOUND EVALUATION

I Just Can't Check My Feet

Why are you delaying the diagnosis of your foot wound? Sometimes people just don't know they have a wound on their foot for various reasons, especially if they can't see the bottom of their foot. You probably don't want to curl your body into a pretzel just so you can simply check your feet every day. There are other ways to make sure your feet get checked regularly. When you go to the doctor, don't be afraid to ask them to take a quick look at the bottom of your feet. It's not enough to just look at the top of your foot, since a lot of wounds occur on the bottom.

Can't stretch out enough to see the bottom of your feet? Maybe you don't have anyone with you regularly to look for you? Try putting a mirror on the floor (but don't leave it there to be walked on) and hold your foot over it to see the bottom of your foot. Don't have a mirror handy? Try using the bottom of a CD, DVD or whatever it is that will reflect an image.

One of the most important things in diagnosing a foot wound is first just learning that you have one. Most wounds aren't found until you have a fever, chills, or they are discovered by accident by someone else. By this time, however, the wound is usually infected.

What Should Skin Look Like?

It's Only Dry Skin

It's not that simple. Most people with diabetes have dry or 'ashy' skin. This is because diabetes affects nerves, which are what feed our sweat glands. If your sweat glands aren't working, then you're not sweating. And no, sweating is NOT a bad thing.

What can you do for your dry skin? Use a cream on your feet and use it every day. Make it a part of your daily routine, whether it's in the morning or just before bed. But, make sure you aren't putting the cream/lotion between your toes because it can get damp in there. Why is this bad? A damp or moist environment in a dark space creates a breeding ground for bacteria.

Corns and Calluses

So what causes foot wounds? Although they seem harmless, calluses can sometimes be painful, and s are actually the leading cause of foot wounds.

What's the difference between a callus and corn? A callus is found on the bottom of feet, while a corn is found on the top of the toes. Corns and calluses are our body's natural way of creating a barrier/protection for any areas of pressure. These can be bad because they are essentially the hardening of skin.

Why care? Well, when skin gets hard, it's not as elastic. If the skin gets too thick, it can crack. So this thick, hard skin needs to be removed. Think of a rubber band: A new rubber band stretches and returns to size with no problems, but a really old rubber band snaps in half when you stretch it. Still don't get it? Picture this: If you held a magnifying glass out in bright sun and the sun shines through it, the light gets focused into a center point. You could take this point of focused light and set something on fire...paper, leaves, and a lot more! Same idea with a callus, but without fire. All the pressure gets placed in one center point and can break down skin. When a callus (or corn) gets trimmed down, the pressure gets evened out again. There are also different types of pads that can be placed in those pressure areas. It's very important to find exactly where the pressure is and to even out the pressure to prevent any injury. It's like when you lay on a bed of nails and it doesn't hurt, but then you step on it with one foot and something bad happens (don't try this at home, but we've all seen this in the movies, right?). Again, it's important to even out pressure.

I Have a Wound, Now What?

So you have a callus (or corn) that continued to get thicker and now you have a wound.

When you get down to the wound after removing all the bad tissue, there are a few things that need to be evaluated. There's something called 'The Ring Effect.' This ring around the wound needs to be removed, so that pressure gets redistributed or evened out. It's important to measure the size of the wound's length, width, and depth. A wound should decrease by 50% in 4 weeks. If this doesn't happen, you will need to change your wound care to help heal the wound faster.

Does the wound undermine? What is undermining? You want to notice if the wound goes deep around the edges. The deeper the wound, the more serious the problem is.

Is there drainage? What color is the drainage? Color is something to pay attention to, as this could really help your doctor to better understand your wound. There are also different types of drainage (thick? clear?).

Is there an odor? Yes this sounds gross, but oddly enough this does also help doctors better understand your wound.

How does the skin around the wound look? Is it red? If you notice a lot of redness, and especially if the redness starts to cover more of your skin, be sure to see a doctor. Redness that quickly covers more skin can be a sign of cellulitis, which is tissue inflammation caused by bad bacteria. Cellulitis needs to be treated with an antibiotic. The skin around the wound can be just as important as the wound itself.

Chronic Wounds

How long has the wound been present? If it's been a long time and the wound hasn't changed, you may need a biopsy. Some people may have a wound present for 20 years and a biopsy is never done. A biopsy can be important with certain chronic wounds.

Ideal Wounds

Did you know that there is an ideal wound? This doesn't mean that wounds are good, it just means that there is a certain type of wound that has the best potential to heal fast.

What does this wound look like and do you have this? The ideal wound has a base that is red, sort of like raw meat (sounds gross, but this is helpful in picturing it). Red or granular tissue is a good sign of healing potential. The ideal wound also has no calluses or really thick skin around the edge of it. Calluses around the edge prevent the wound edges from moving closer together and closing.

The 'Special Event Wound'

This is really exactly what it sounds like. You had to go to dinner, wedding, date, or whatever and you had to wear a different pair of shoes than you normally do. Before you even make it home in time to throw those shoes off, you find a blister. Blisters are the next big cause of wounds. Blisters contain fluid. Once the blister breaks open, it can be slow to heal and can develop into an ulcer.

What a Warm Foot Means for Wound Healing

Doesn't a warm foot mean a healthy foot? Usually yes, but sometimes a foot is just too warm. A foot that is too warm can sometimes be a sign of what doctors call a 'Charcot' foot. 'Charcot' is pronounced like 'shar-coh', and it's not really just a fancy French-sounding name. It's actually a type of foot where the foot heats up and then collapses over time.

A temperature stat is one device that measures the temperature on the bottom of your foot. There is a new fabric on the market today that can change color with the heat from your hand, which is a similar idea as the temperature board. When there is an area of increased temperature (or pressure), it changes color. A wound always develops in an area of increased temperature, such as with the 'Charcot foot.'

But I Still Can't See My Foot

No excuses! There's the old saying, "Where there is a will, there is a way." There is a casual and formal way to check your feet. The casual way includes having a friend, loved one, or visiting nurse to check your feet/wound every day. Again, you can and should use a mirror to check if you have no one around to help you out. Can't see that far? You can try using your phone to take a picture or video of your wound. This will also be helpful to your healthcare provider who can see how the wound has changed over time. The formal way to check your feet is, of course, to see a doctor, but most importantly, just have your feet inspected.

STEP 4: BONE AND PRESSURE EVALUATION

How Does a Wound Develop?

You're probably getting a wound due to a bony prominence or from increased pressure on the bottom of your foot.

But you're not walking on the wound, right? You can deny it all day, but your wound says it all. Your wound will show how much you've really been walking. However, it's also very difficult to get pressure off of these wounds.

What risk factors are there for developing a foot wound? An area of increased pressure is a major risk factor for developing a wound. Where are the bony prominences? Bony prominences are areas where bone is obviously bigger than it should be, or causing pain with wearing shoes or walking. Where are the high-pressure areas? A classic sign of a high-pressure area is the presence of a callus (as we discussed earlier). Again, calluses and corns can really slow wound healing.

Checking for Areas of Pressure

There is a special mat called a Pressure Mat, or a Harris Mat that works in a similar way as some duplicate checks. When you write this check, the writing transfers to the carbon copy of the check. This mat basically develops a carbon copy of the bottom of your foot and can help identify where your areas of pressure are.

Certain types of feet are more likely to develop high-pressure areas. Also, as we age, the fat on the bottom of our feet gets redistributed. This means we have less fat in the areas we really need padding at. Some people will joke, "Well the fat moves from the foot to somewhere else." Yes, but this doesn't mean it all went to your hips or waist. If the fat on the bottom of your feet isn't in the areas of high-pressure, then your skin is almost in direct contact with the bone and is more likely to develop a wound.

So, where are these pressure areas?

There are certainly common areas of high-pressure on the bottom of your feet, including right below your big toe joint, the heel, the 5th (small) toe, and sometimes under the center of your foot (if your foot has collapsed in the center). Once you've identified any high-pressure areas, you can then 'off-load' these areas with special pads and/or shoes.

Are high-pressure areas only on the bottom of feet? Pressure areas can also develop on the top or sides of feet, including the side of the big toe (often called a 'pinch callus'). A pinch callus develops because you don't have enough movement in the big toe joint. Motion has to happen somewhere, so it occurs in another joint. Doctors like to call this 'hallux limitus' or 'hallux rigidus.'

Other Pressure Areas

Some people get wounds at the very tip of their toes due to hammertoes. Here's a tip: If you can take this curled toe and straighten it out, this is a 'flexible hammertoe.' If you try to straighten the toe and just can't, this is a 'rigid hammertoe.' When you walk, the top or tip of this curled toe can rub against the inside of your shoes and can create a corn or wound on either the top or tip of the toe. Flexible hammertoes can typically be treated with padding, but sometimes surgery is needed to treat the rigid type. Sometimes the tendon on the bottom of the toe needs to be cut, which can be easily done (even right in the office). Cutting the tendon will straighten the toe, then removing pressure on the tip of the toe.

Sounds easy, right? It's important to remember that by correcting a hammertoe, it is also possible for pressure to be transferred to another area, another toe, etc.

Sometimes wounds just can't be treated with special dressings or shoes. Because these pressure areas can cause slow to heal or non-healing wounds, sometimes the problem needs to be corrected with surgery to remove some of the bone or to help create more motion at a joint.

Big Bad Causes

What area common causes for high-pressure areas or bony prominences? Combine the foot with the type of shoes that are being worn. If shoes aren't appropriate for your foot type, your foot can rub in certain areas that may not necessarily be painful, but can create pressure, calluses, or even blisters. Common problems that can cause rubbing in shoes include hallux limitus/rigidus, bunions, and hammertoes. For example, if you have a bunion, sometimes the bone can rub against the inside of your shoes and you will develop redness or even a wound at that area. It can be difficult to find the right shoe gear because sometimes the most appropriate or comfortable shoes for your feet aren't always the most attractive. It's also important to either find shoes with padding in the right areas for your feet or to remember to add padding in those areas.

How Flexible Are You?

What does your flexibility have to do with bones and wound healing? Well, if you don't have enough flexibility at a joint, pressure gets transferred somewhere else. Some people have a tight heel cord, which is a condition called 'equinus.' If you have equinus, your foot doesn't flex past 90 degrees, which creates more pressure on the bottom of your forefoot. Some people can treat this with regular stretching exercises while others need surgery to lengthen the Achilles tendon. Both of these treatments are designed to help the foot flex past 90 degrees.

It's important to remember that with slow-healing wounds, sometimes it's not the wound itself. Slow or non-healing wounds can also be due to problems with nerves, muscles, or tendons, all which work together.

Let's Talk About Charcot

Remember that fancy French term we discussed earlier? A Charcot foot is when you break your foot and don't know it. But that's ridiculous, how can you break your foot and not know it? Yes, it's possible. With Charcot, you don't have any feeling in your feet (neuropathy). A Charcot foot can become red, hot, and swollen, and if you keep walking on it, it will continue to break. It's not unusual to have a lack of pain with this, and it often gets misdiagnosed or mislabeled as an infection. This foot type can continue to break down and get to a point where the foot looks like a 'rocker-bottom.' This is similar to the idea of a rocking chair. A wound can develop on the bottom of this "rocker" and can be very challenging to heal. It is VERY important to reduce the pressure through padding, appropriate shoe gear, or even surgery.

Things to remember: Make sure you're always asking, "What's causing my wound?" There are a lot of factors that can contribute to the cause of a wound, and it's important to identify all of the possibilities so that you can heal your wound fast.

STEP 5: NERVES AND FEELING EVALUATION

How Neuropathy Affects Wound Healing

Have you ever had a papercut on your finger and then avoided using that finger for a while? It hurts right? You protect it, put a band-aid on it and probably have a little pain for a couple hours. The same thing would apply if you had a cut on the bottom of your foot, as you'd probably protect it, or maybe walk a little differently due to the pain.

Diabetics can lose this important gift of pain. Neuropathy is the lack of sensation or pain. Why would anyone call pain a gift? Pain protects and helps us. Without pain, you'd continue walking on your foot when something is wrong. Pain is our body's red flag that something isn't right. The biggest difficulty doctors have when treating a wound is that people will keep walking on it because it doesn't hurt.

Long ago, there were different groups of people referred to as 'lepers.' With leprosy, people lost feeling and sensation in their hands and feet. This lack of feeling became so bad that they could cut off fingers or toes without knowing it, and would die from the bleeding. You could have good blood flow and no other health problems, but you can't protect yourself if you can't feel anything.

Neuropathy From the Beginning

What is neuropathy? 'Neuro' means nerve and 'path' means injury, so neuropathy is injury to a nerve. Let's start at the spinal cord. In your spinal cord, there are a lot of nerves that go out to all the different areas of your body. The farther these nerves are from your spinal cord, the smaller they get. The farther and smaller these nerves are, the more affected they are by your blood sugar.

Every nerve has two blood vessels following it side-by-side, because nerves are very dependent on blood flow and circulation. Losing blood flow to a nerve for even a few seconds can kill the nerve. A good example of this is when infants are born with the spinal cord wrapped around their neck. This can cause brain death because blood flow to their brain is blocked. Nerves are the most sensitive organ in the human body to blood flow. Nerves need good, healthy blood flow. If a nerve is injured, it takes a long time to heal.

Why Sugar is Bad for Nerves

With diabetes, the blood vessels that run with each nerve have a lot of sugar in them. Nerves are bathed in blood so when sugar is too high, the nerves can swell. When the nerves swell, their conduction becomes affected. Nerve impulses start to decrease or slow. Eventually these impulses will decrease so much that they will completely stop. However, the impulses don't just stop quickly. Let's think about the lights in your house during a bad storm. The lights will typically start to flicker for a bit then eventually go out. This is a similar idea as to your nerves. The "flickering" in your nerves will usually start as painful tingling or burning sensations. Again, pain is OK because this is your warning signal.

There are medications that can help with the pain, but it's very difficult to heal nerves. The best thing you can do to control your neuropathy is to control your blood sugar. There are medications that can help with nerve function, but a lot of them are still being tested, and there are, of course, no guarantee that your nerve function will ever return to normal.

It's important to know that diabetes is not the only reason a person can have neuropathy, although it is the most common cause. There can be a lot of other causes including long-term alcohol use, or even certain medications.

Testing My Nerves

If you're in the beginning stages of neuropathy, you should regularly see your podiatrist, even if you don't currently have a wound. It's important to prevent any problems or disease. We still go to the dentist for check-ups even if we don't have any obvious problems, right? We go to the eye doctor because he/she can see things that your family doctor can't see.

Your podiatrist can evaluate the level at which you've lost feeling in your feet. This is simply done by using something called a monofilament. A monofilament is a thin piece of plastic that looks like fishing line and is used to push on different areas of your feet. It's a good sign if you can feel all of the different areas that are touched on your feet. Callused areas of your feet will make it more difficult for you to feel this wire. If you can't feel some of the areas, then you've probably lost 'protective sensation,' or the ability to detect pressure. This is bad because if you step on something, you probably won't know it, which puts you at a higher risk for developing a foot wound or ulcer. Painful wounds tend to heal faster than non-painful wounds. Again, if you have a foot wound that doesn't hurt, you're probably going to keep walking on it.

Vibratory sensation is another sign that should be checked. In your spinal cord, you have different tracts or lines that feel touch, hot or cold sensations, and sharp or dull sensations. A device called a tuning fork is used to check for the sensation of vibration. The tuning fork is hit so that it vibrates, then is placed on different areas of your foot. If both you and your tester can feel when it stops, then your vibration sensation is OK. There is a problem when you can't feel the vibration and your tester still can. This means that you have some beginning signs of neuropathy, which don't always have to be painful.

Your reflexes can also be tested. If your reflexes aren't good, you're at an increased risk for developing a wound on the bottom of your foot.

Anything else? There's one more test called the 'vibration perception threshold testing,' which is a vibration test, but is more costly than others. You will find that some doctors do not use it. Don't be afraid to ask your doctor how to test for this.

My Wound Won't Heal Fast

Again, pain is a good thing because it's our body's warning signal. Neuropathy, or lack of feeling is one of the leading causes of why wounds don't heal. One of the major challenges people often have is that they have places to go, jobs to perform, or people to take care of, but walking on the wound will just delay or prevent healing.

How do you know how much you're really walking? Try and keep track of how many steps you take in a day. You'd be surprised how much distance you can cover just by walking all over your house several times a day.

Things to remember: Control your blood sugar and take care of your nerves. Once your nerves go bad, you probably can't go back. Also, monitor how much you've really been walking. Your trips to the bathroom, kitchen, bed, and couch all add up to a much greater distance than you'd think. Lack of feeling and walking a lot of miles really won't help with healing your wound fast.

STEP 6: WOUND DEBRIDEMENT AND SURGERY

Wound Treatment and Evaluation

How is your wound currently being treated? Has it ever been treated? Should you even bother to seek treatment? Why does your wound need treatment? Do you just have a callus?

Well, remember earlier that calluses have a 60% increase in pressure under that area. If your callus is trimmed down regularly, you'll be able to get a better look at that skin under it. There are people that will go to a doctor to have their callus trimmed down, their doctor will find a wound, and people will say, "Well the doctor *gave* me that wound." That wound was already there. Your body made the callus to protect it.

So calluses cause wounds, but they protect too?

Well, yes. For example, when you do a lot of work using your hands, maybe working in the yard or using a shovel, you'll develop calluses on your hands. Calluses reduce the friction force, but if you *overuse* your hands, you'll develop a blister. This is the same way it works in the foot. When you have an area of high pressure in the foot (bony prominence, tight heel cord, etc.), this pressure can produce a blister, callus, or even a wound. If the callus continues to get bigger, something will have to happen to it. It will have to either fall off or crack and develop a wound. If you wait that long to go to the doctor and have it treated, don't be surprised if it's painful. With the right conditions, sometimes an infection can begin and will need to be 'relieved.'

But don't let it get this far, just have it trimmed and inspected regularly.

The most common type of wound seen on the bottom or side of the foot is a wound with a callus on top of it or around it. The callus creates an 'edge effect' (remember this from an earlier section?). This is when there appears to be a ring around the ulcer, which will often cover up the ulcer and make it look healed.

Calluses will Fool You

Picture this: If there's an avalanche in a cave, everything will be covered over. If you're inside the cave, the cave is still there even though it's completely covered on the outside. But, you'd think it was a solid, stable area if you were looking at it from outside the cave. Same idea with a wound: the wound is deep, but the callus is covering it and so it looks healed.

So the callus will stop as soon as you stop putting pressure on that area, right? Not exactly. Skin has some memory to it, so a callus won't magically disappear if you stop putting pressure on it for one day.

When treating a wound, what you remove from it is more important than what you put on. What does this mean? There are A LOT of different wound care products out there and we all hope for one product to be the magic cure-all. But first, it is most important to *remove* something.

So, What Gets Removed?

First, you want to remove any excess pressure on the area by using a special shoe, avoiding walking on it, adding special padding to your shoe, and removing any 'bad' skin. 'Bad' skin is any of the dead tissue on top of the wound that doesn't bleed. Don't be afraid of a little bleeding, as bleeding means that you'll be able to heal the wound under the right conditions. If the tissue doesn't bleed, then it's not living tissue and is tissue that's either callused or infected. Your doctor hasn't accidentally cut you and made you bleed. Your doctor is *hoping* you bleed and you should too because, again, bleeding means your wound can heal.

So, what should the wound look like? As we reviewed earlier, the edges should be healthy tissue that bleeds and the base should be red (like red meat). This is the type of tissue your body needs to heal the wound.

A Living Example

There's a person I know who is missing his big toe, and so all the pressure that's supposed to be under his big toe goes under the second toe. So, he has a callus under his second toe from all the pressure. He has regular check-ups and wears special shoes. There was a time when he went on a trip for 3-4 months and when he returned, the callus had a wound underneath it.

Again, it's very important to have your calluses trimmed down. Sometimes when a callus is trimmed down and has a wound under it, the wound might appear bigger.

But My Wound Doesn't Look Red and Beefy

So what happens when your wound isn't red and healthy looking? What if you see muscle or tendon, or even bone? Well, this changes your treatment. First, your wound has to heal over the bone, tendon, or muscle (whichever is exposed). Second, any yellow tissue has to be turned into red (healthy) tissue. These can be done in several different ways.

Sometimes a wound is infected and the longer your wound is open, the more likely it is to develop an infection. It can look red (a healthy red will look different from an infected red), swollen, or be painful. Infection is bad, so this is why it's so important to heal the wound fast. Many infections lead to amputation and so the faster you heal them, the easier it is to avoid an infection.

What to Know About Cultures

Cultures can tell you a lot about a wound, but they can also fool you. A lot of people who take wound cultures and don't usually see a lot of wounds will just take a quick sample from tissue on the top of the wound. Samples from the top of a wound really aren't the best cultures. Our skin normally has a lot of contaminants on it, so samples from the top of a wound may give a false idea of what's really in your wound. The best culture is taken when you see healthy red tissue, *after* you've gotten rid of all the bad tissue.

If you do have an infection, there are many medications you can take to help get rid of the infection. There are both oral and intravenous antibiotics available, which are prescribed based on how bad your infection is and what your cultures reveal.

When Your Bone is Infected

Sometimes a wound starts out small or not very deep, then gets infected and becomes deep. There are mainly two options and the first is intravenous antibiotics for 6-8 weeks. The second option is to simply have surgery to have the infected bone removed. Some people have wounds that heal and then come back, and sometimes even come back with a vengeance. One of the biggest reasons why the wound keeps coming back is because the bone was infected and never completely healed. If this is the case, the infected bone will have to be removed.

When Your Wound is Really Old

Sometimes wounds can actually transform into a type of cancer. When you have a wound that's been open or just not healing for a long time, it could have something doctors call a 'malignant transformation.' If you have a wound that hasn't healed for years, you should have a biopsy taken. It's important to make sure your wound isn't being infected by something else and that there isn't a 'malignant transformation' of that wound.

Things to remember: Please don't take a kitchen knife and trim your callus yourself. Please don't do any bathroom surgery. For all the ladies out there (and men, too), sometimes nail salons will trim calluses. It would be best to skip this service because their tools aren't always clean. Please see a doctor to be treated and monitored regularly. If you have a wound, it needs treatment. It's important to get rid of excess pressure and bad tissue in order to help heal your wound fast.

STEP 7: WOUND DRESSINGS AND GRAFTS

Wound Dressings

If you have a wound, you really shouldn't be walking around with the wound exposed to everything around you. The more things your wound is exposed to, the greater the risk of infection. It should really be covered and protected. until it is healed or has a callus over it.

Once your wound has been debrided (or cleaned up) in the office, you need to look at the wound. Sometimes, the wound can have a biofilm over it.

What are Biofilms?

In a wound, your body is producing different types of chemicals (growth hormones, etc.) to try to help heal the wound. Sometimes, there's a thin clear film that can develop over the wound (sort of like soap scum in a tub or sink). Biofilm slows the wound in its healing process because it slows down the growth hormones and growth process. This biofilm needs to be removed by either being scrubbed or scraped away.

Why Cover Wounds?

Wound dressings (or coverings) are used to protect the wound from infection, but also to provide padding from trauma/injury and to collect any type of drainage from the wound. The type of dressing will depend on its purpose.

The Right Dressing

So how do you know what type of dressing is right for you? Well there isn't always a "right" dressing. It's probably easiest to think of a wound as wet or dry. If the wound is wet, you need to dry it out. If the wound is dry, you need to moisten it. Simply putting gauze in and taking it out provides mechanical debridement, meaning that each time you take the gauze out some of the bad tissue will be removed. Again, what you put on the wound is not as important as what is removed (callus, bad tissue, and biofilm AKA "soap scum").

Determining what dressing to use is simpler than it seems. Take a look at your wound. If your wound is draining a lot, then you need something to absorb the drainage. One dressing used for this is made of seaweed, its called an 'alginate.' This absorbs much more than you think it will. If your wound is deep AND draining a lot, then a foam type dressing would be better because a foam can be put inside the wound and will absorb. If you have a wound that is more black and dry (doctors call this 'necrotic' or 'gangrenous'), you want to make it more moist/wet. This would need something called a 'hydrogel,' which looks pretty similar to the gel you would use in your hair. Hydrogels keep the wound area moist. If you have a wound with healthy red tissue, then you want a dressing that will help promote 'epithelialization' (i.e. healing). There are several different dressings that can be used, including the hydrogel.

There are also challenging wounds that have yellow, fibrous tissue. With these, you want dressings that will absorb any drainage, but also help transform that bad yellow tissue into healthy red. We want to transform this wound from 'fibrous' to 'granular.'

If you have an infected wound, an iodine or a silver dressing typically works best. These dressings have antibacterial properties, which can help get rid of the infection and help the wound heal faster.

Who Changes the Dressings

It's not necessarily about *who* changes the dressing. Sometimes it's difficult for you to see your doctor frequently to have your dressings changed, especially if your dressing needs to be changed daily or even several times a day. Sometimes it's hard for you to get out of your house for different reasons. Some people with certain criteria can have people visit your house to do these dressing changes for you or even instruct a family member on how to do this. It's best to have someone change the dressing for you so they can see how the wound has changed. Have this person take note of how the wound has changed in size, color, drainage, and smell/odor.

Remember, just because your dressing gets changed regularly, it won't magically heal if you're walking on it constantly.

There is another type of passive therapy called a 'bioengineered skin substitute.' There are two main ones used, Apligraf and Dermagraft. These are both skin substitutes that can only be placed on wounds with that healthy, beefy red tissue to help heal the wound faster. These are for the person who wouldn't be a good candidate for a skin graft, but still wants to heal the wound faster. These carry growth hormones and healing components to help form a covering over the top of the wound. Think of this as a sort of scaffolding, where your own skin can heal over the top of the scaffold. Your wound may require several applications of Apligraf or Dermagraft.

Are You Right for a 'Bioengineered Skin Substitute'?

Unfortunately in the US, this is determined by your insurance. But insurance will usually cover these because they greatly reduce the healing time of foot wounds. Wounds are costly, and skin substitutes help heal wounds fast.

If your wound heals anyway, why does it matter how quickly it heals? The faster your wound heals, the faster you can continue on with your life. With an open wound, you are less likely to walk and exercise, and then tend to gain weight. The more weight you gain, the harder it is to control your blood sugar. A wound on your foot can make it difficult for you to drive, play with your kids or grandkids, or simply live your life.

Guidelines of Healing

Here it is: If you have a foot wound for over 4 weeks that doesn't decrease in size by 50%, then you qualify for some type of synthetic skin covering. You will have to find a doctor who is comfortable with this and has experience in applying these skin substitutes.

How will you know if your wound has decreased? Upon your initial visit and every visit to your doctor, make sure your wound gets measured. Some people even like to take pictures of their wounds to help monitor how their wound has changed (or not changed).

Active Therapies

Everything reviewed until now have all been passive therapies. So then what are active therapies? One example is a Negative Pressure Wound Therapy or VAC assisted closure. This is basically putting foam in your wound, then putting a mini vacuum on top, and sucking all the drainage out. A constant suction (or pulling on the wound) will increase the blood flow to the wound and also reduce any swelling, which helps heal your wound fast.

These "vacuums" can't be walked on, especially if it's on the bottom of your foot. However, if you've had daily or several times a day dressing changes, these will require less frequent changes. The big challenge with the VAC assisted closure is that it can cause the sides of the wound to be damp. If the skin is damp, it can get what doctors call 'macerated' (meaning tissues will get soft and white). This is the same idea as when you stay in the bathtub, shower, or pool too long and you notice your fingers turning really soft, white, and wrinkly.

Another therapy is Regranex, which is a platelet-derived growth factor. Platelets are the healing components in your blood and can help the wound heal faster. An important note is that Regranex isn't always covered by insurance.

Hyperbaric oxygen is yet another therapy that is used in healing foot wounds fast. This is an advanced treatment and not all doctors do this. You need to speak with your doctor to determine the best treatment for healing your wound fast.

Things to Remember: Visit a doctor to figure out the best dressing for your wound. It's important to remove bad tissue and pressure from your wound. Also, make sure you monitor your wound each time your dressing is changed, so that you and your doctor can together figure out the best way to heal your wound fast.

STEP 8: SHOES AND OFF-LOADING

Off-Loading Your Wound

You should know by now that if you have a foot wound, you really shouldn't be walking on it, right? And that if you don't have the gift of feeling (so you've got neuropathy), any cut or wound on your foot won't hurt? Well the problem with having neuropathy AND a diabetic foot wound is that you don't experience pain; you won't be aware of any foot problems. By far, many doctors find the number one reason that foot wounds don't heal is due to increased pressure on the wound. Also, are you following the recommendations given to you?

But we can't really entirely blame patients (you) for why your wound isn't healing. We understand that you have a life: things to do, a home to tend to, kids to drive around, and people to care for. We know you don't have time to wait and watch the skin grow over your wound, because this could take months.

A Living Example

I had a patient who had a wound for many, many months. She had these special shoes that were designed to help offload the area, meaning they redistributed pressure so it wasn't all focused at the wound. With further questioning (yes, the truth will come out), I quickly learned that she only wore these special shoes when she visited my office. Sure, she stayed home a lot, but wore regular bedroom slippers instead of these special shoes. But as discussed earlier, you'd be surprised to learn how much you actually walk around your home. Not wearing the right shoes can create a real challenge when trying to heal your foot wound. Remember, your feet carry the weight of your entire body...so treat them well! Nothing will change unless you help in making a change!

Now of course, everything is important: blood sugar control, good blood flow, and checking that there's no deeper infection. Making sure all of these factors are OK won't matter if you don't take the pressure off of your wound, because it still won't heal if there's pressure

Track Your Walking

Get a pedometer, a device to help you track exactly how much you're really walking. A pedometer will really keep you honest about how much you're walking, including inside your house!

So How Do You Get Pressure Off a Wound and Heal it?

Here's the plan: You're going to lie in bed all day for 3 months. But that would be impossible, right? So how can you realistically do this?

Realistic Treatments for Pressure Relief

Ever heard of a roll-about? A roll-about is similar to a walker, but you put one knee up on a rest instead of on the ground. Then, you simply roll around. The only problem with this is that the opposite foot is on the ground and bearing more weight than usual.

Then of course there's the wheelchair. You certainly won't be putting any pressure on your feet sitting in a wheelchair. The only problem with a wheelchair is that it requires a decent amount of upper body (arm) strength to be able to use it by yourself. The same problem occurs with using crutches.

Remember that when you have a wound or a callus with a wound underneath it, there's a 60% increase in pressure at that area? This 60% increase is like a magnifying glass, focusing all the pressure in one area. Some people will have more than one pressure area and it's important to spread this pressure out evenly.

What Happens When Your Foot Has More than One Pressure Area?

Getting pressure off of one area is tough, but two areas is even more challenging. So how do you do this? The best way of doing this is with something called a Total Contact Cast (TCC). It's a cast with minimal padding and it's totally in contact with your leg and foot, so it transfers the pressure from one area to the entire leg and foot. The only problem with this is that you have to keep it on for one week, so you won't be able to monitor your wound. People with infected wounds can't get a TCC, because you won't want to cover an infected wound for a week without checking it frequently. People with heavily draining wounds probably shouldn't get a TCC either, because then all the drainage would collect in the cast. Also, if this cast isn't applied correctly and you have neuropathy, it could create new wounds. Not all doctors like or feel comfortable using this type of cast.

The TCC has great success rates when applied correctly. It also allows you to walk around (but you still can't run a marathon). The TCC reduces pressure on the wound by about 80-90%, allowing for the wound to heal.

Other options for getting pressure off of an area include:

A Removable Cast Walker is a big boot that help reduces pressure on the bottom of your foot. It moves like a rocking chair at the bottom, allowing you to flow and roll through your step.

The 'half shoe' or an Ortho Wedge Shoe. This is like if you took a shoe, cut it in half, then left either the front or back on depending on the location of the wound. For example, if the wound is in the front of your foot, you'll only put on the back part of the shoe so that you're only putting pressure on the heel. If you have a heel wound, you can only put pressure on the front. Be sure when wearing this type of shoe you don't push off the front of the foot. This will defeat the purpose of the shoe.

A surgical shoe, or a 'flatbed' shoe, doesn't bend and so it helps reduce pressure on the bottom of the foot. Sometimes, your doctor will have to adjust the shoe and add a cutout or foam padding based on your specific wound.

Felt padding. This is padding that is added under the wound to off-load the area of ulceration. This can be removed to change the dressing daily and then taped in the area again. It tends to stay in the proper location better than the surgical shoe with padding.

It's important to be careful when you first start using any of these shoes. Your hip level will be different and will affect how you walk. You may have to find a shoe with a small heel to wear on your good foot in order to balance yourself out. Also, using one of these devices still doesn't mean you can continue walking a lot.

Are You Wearing the Right Shoe Size?

A lot of people with diabetes are absolutely certain they know what size shoes they wear. You've been that shoe size your entire life right? Well, in diabetics and especially in females after they age and/or have children, there's a hormone (called relaxin) that relaxes your ligaments and so your shoe size can increase over time.

Your shoe size can also change due to a bunion, hammertoe, or other problems. It's important to be professionally measured to find your correct shoe size. Wrong shoe sizes can create wounds! So if you already know that the shoes you're wearing right now are the wrong size, *please* get rid of them right now! Also, regularly check that there is nothing inside the shoe, such as a coin, rock, or even a toy.

But I Have to Work

At what point should you stop working and really stay off of your feet? A situation when this would be important is if you've had a wound for a really long time and it's gotten infected. You should really consider whether working or keeping your leg is more important to you.

Again, offloading is extremely important, but it's not the only thing. Remember, there are 9 total steps in healing wounds fast. We've reviewed the importance of controlling blood sugar, having good blood flow, reducing bony prominence pressure, adjusting for neuropathy, having the right wound dressing and wound care. But all of these *don't matter* if you don't get the pressure off of your feet. This step was left until now because it's THE most important aspect of healing your foot wound. After the wound is healed, you can fix bony prominences or the shoes you're wearing.

This course was designed to help in healing wounds fast and that's the goal. However, wounds heal slowly, that's why I'm giving you all of the tips to help heal your wound fast. Searching for information online can be overwhelming because there's just too much information out there, so that's why I've summarized the most important tips. You'll also have access to my handout that will allow you to see how you're doing in healing your wound fast. This will help you do your own diabetic exam, and will be especially helpful if you don't have access to the care of a podiatrist.

My ultimate goal is to have a world without unnecessary amputations. The last step in this series is how to prevent recurrence. Why is this important if you've now healed your foot wound? Because once you've had a wound, you're at a much greater risk of developing another wound.

STEP 9: PREVENTING RECURRENCE AND OTHER COMPLICATIONS

So you've managed to heal your foot wound fast. What happens now? Well, you want to prevent another wound because once you've had a wound you're more likely to get another one. Here are some tips on what to do now:

Continue to check your feet daily!

Get a diabetic foot exam. How often this happens will depend on your blood flow, foot type, and sensation. You might have to get an exam anywhere from every 2 months to once a year.

Podiatrists don't just trim your nails and calluses so your feet will look good. They do this to help prevent wounds.

Get diabetic shoes. They help prevent wounds.

Wear your diabetic shoes at home. Wear SOMETHING that will protect your feet if you bump into things.

Your healthcare team is made up of people that work together to help you stay healthy. It can include a blood flow doctor, infectious disease doctor, skin doctor, physical therapist, pedorthist (shoe specialist), cast technician, visiting home nurse, dietician, endocrinologist, primary care or family doctor, kidney doctor, eye doctor, and/or brain doctor.

So What's Next?

So you've managed to heal your wound fast...but now how do you prevent recurrence? The single most important tip I can provide you with is to look at and inspect your feet *daily*. Look at the top, between the toes to make sure there is no dampness or moisture, and at the bottom of your feet. Some patients have what is called the 'dunlop disease'...you know, they have a big belly and it 'dun lopped' over their belt buckle and can't see their feet! Some people have back problems or painful joints that don't allow them to see their feet. Have someone, *anyone*, look at your feet for cuts, blisters, or dampness.

When you first learn that you have diabetes, it's easy to blame someone else. But you have to take control and take care of yourself and your diabetes.

When Do I Get a Diabetic Foot Exam?

It's also important to have a 'comprehensive diabetic foot exam.' This really includes an evaluation of overall general health, blood flow, skin, musculoskeletal system, and shoes. Recommendations will be made to you afterwards. Dr. Bolton developed these recommendations, which have since been adopted by the American Diabetes Association.

There are 3 risk categories. A risk of 0 means you have NO problems with blood flow, foot deformity, or neuropathy. You should visit a doctor once a year to have your feet checked and cared for. A risk of 1 means you have neuropathy (or bad feeling) and/or a deformity. You should be seen twice a year or every 6 months. You may also need different shoes or to consider having the deformity corrected. A risk of 2 means you may have poor blood flow, swelling, and/or a lack of feeling. You should be seen every 2-3 months for a check-up. You should also be wearing the right shoes and you may even need to see a blood flow doctor.

Why 2-3 months?

If you fall into the risk 2 group, you may be seeing a podiatrist every couple of months. You will have your nails or calluses trimmed (remember, to reduce high pressure areas) to prevent wounds in the first place.

The last and worst category to fall into is 3. This is for people who have had a history of a wound or an amputation. If you fall into this group, you should really be seeing a blood flow doctor.

Do I Need Diabetic Shoes?

What is a diabetic shoe? It's an 'extra-depth' shoe that's a little deeper than a normal shoe. It has special inserts that are put into the shoe. There are two different types of inserts that are used to reduce the sliding-around motion (friction) of your foot in the shoe. You have to be measured for these shoes, so don't assume that your shoe size will be the same as your regular shoes, because you're probably wearing the wrong size. If you have neuropathy and your shoe *feels* like it fits, it's probably too small. If you wear a shoe that's too small, you'll feel the pressure of it and think this means that the shoe fits. Your shoe also shouldn't feel too big or 'flop around.' A correct fit might feel *a little* big if you're neuropathic.

Insurance companies cover diabetic shoes because wounds are expensive. If they can give out 300 pairs of diabetic shoes and prevent one wound, then that's a good thing. Bad shoes cause a lot of foot problems and wounds, even if they are worn for only a couple hours.

Other People Who Can Get Diabetic Shoes

People who have a history of amputation of a toe or foot, a previous wound, calluses that are almost wounds, neuropathy with calluses, bad blood flow, or a foot deformity (bunion, hammertoe, bony prominence) can also get diabetic shoes. There are two types of shoes: over the counter and custom shoes. You should see a specialist to see which type is right for you.

You should get 3 pairs of diabetic shoes each year. It's best to switch them every 4 months. If it helps, write the date on the bottom of the shoe each time you put a new one on so you'll know how long you've been wearing that pair.

But I Don't Wear Shoes at Home

It's really best to wear shoes while walking around at home too, but sometimes it's not practical. The shoe brand Crocs make diabetic clogs that can be worn at home to help protect your feet if you accidentally bump or stub your toes. It's important to wear a shoe that will protect your feet. Don't go barefoot at home. Also, wearing regular sandals or flip-flops during summer is dangerous and can create foot problems...so be careful!

Who is On My Healthcare Team?

Who makes up your healthcare team depends on every person's needs. If you have a wound, you should be seeing a podiatrist who can evaluate and debride (or clean up) the wound and give the right dressings or medications. Some podiatrists work in a wound care clinic, which would also be a great place to find care. Other people you may also need to see include:

A circulation or blood flow doctor who will be able to look at any changes in your blood flow. Blood flow is needed for healing wounds!

Infectious disease or skin doctor who can look at the skin around the wound and look for any infection.

Physical therapist to help with walking or balancing problems. This person is especially important if you feel unstable or if you trip and fall a lot.

You may need a pedorthist to help find and fit you with the right shoe.

Cast tech, or someone to take off and apply your Total Contact Cast.

Nurse or an aide to visit your home and help with wound care.

Dietician to help find foods that are OK for diabetics to eat.

Endocrinologist and primary care doctor to help monitor your diabetes and blood sugar.

Kidney doctor (nephrologist) to work with you because diabetes affects your kidneys.

Eye doctor, because your eyes can also be affected in diabetes. Retinopathy is a disease that affects the small blood vessels in your eyes and can worsen your eyesight.

<u>Brain</u> doctor (neurologist) because poorly controlled diabetes affects everything!

You should also have a place to go in case of an <u>emergency</u>. If you have diabetes AND neuropathy, you are at a high risk of this happening.

YOUTUBE LINKS

Here you will find a compilation of videos that go over the 9 steps to wound healing.

https://youtu.be/KZPcgtYf49M

TELEPHONE INFORMATION

For those that do not have access to the internet here is a phone number that you can call to hear information about wound healing. Just enter in the appropriate codes to hear the topics that mean the most to you. This is especially good for those who are visually impaired.

Dial-in Number: (641) 715-3800

Code: 32299#

100 - Introduction to healing your foot wound (12:58 min)

101 - How blood sugar and nutrition can affect wound healing (12:17 min)

102 - How blood flow and swelling affect wound healing (13:52 min)

103 - How to evaluate your wound properly (13:51 min)

104 – How to reduce pressure under your wound (14:04 min)

105 - How poor feeling can affect wound healing (13:20 min)

106 - Why debriding the wound and surgery is sometimes necessary to heal wounds (13.39 min)

107 - How to choose a dressing for your wound and when grafts are needed (14:42 min)

108 - How to off-load your wound and when you can start wearing a normal shoe again (16:53 min)

WOUND PROGRESS TRACKING SHEET

Instructions: This sheet can be copied and brought to your doctor's visits to track the size of your foot wound.

Doctor: _____

Ulcer Treatment Tool

Diagnosis:_____

Cause:_____

Next Appointment: 1 2 3 4 6 8 Weeks

Infection: No   Yes - Antibiotic _____

Wound Dressing: _____

Off-Loading: _____

Homework: _____

Next Steps: _____

Wound Size Tracking Tool

Date: Size:
Notes:

Date: Size:
Notes:

Date: Size:
Notes:

Date: Size:
Notes:

Date: Size:
Notes:

Step Tracking (Track how many steps per day)

What worked with your treatment up to this point?

What did not work?

What would you do differently?

WOUND AUDIT

Instructions

Here are a series of questions that will help you understand more about your foot wound to make sure you are doing the best you can to heal it quickly.

Please note that the questions are organized to follow the information in this book. For more information on each question please visit the appropriate section and review the information in that specific step by reading that information.

If you are seeing a doctor for treatment you can fill this out and bring it to the doctor's office.

Step 1 - Blood Sugar and Nutrition

Many factors affect the healing of your foot wound, including your general health, nutrition, and keeping your diabetes under control.

Here you can learn more about how this affects your wound healing.

How long have you had your foot wound?

> Less than a month
>
> 1-2 months
>
> 3-12 months
>
> Over a year
>
> I don't know

Do you have diabetes?

Yes

No

Not sure

What was your last Hemoglobin A1C?

A normal number is 7 or below.

Under 7

7-9

Over 9

I don't know

Do you smoke?

Smoking can affect and slow down wound healing.

Yes

No

I have quit - Congratulations!!

Do you take a multivitamin?

Many people with foot wounds don't get all the nutrients needed, and a multivitamin can help.

Yes

No

Do you get enough protein?

When you have a foot wound extra protein is needed to help the wound heal.

> Yes
>
> No
>
> I don't know?

Can you feel your foot pulses?

> Yes
>
> No
>
> I don't know?

Step 2 - Blood Flow and Swelling

Here are a number of questions relating to the circulation in your feet.

Do you have swelling?

Swelling can slow down healing and needs to be controlled.

> Yes
>
> No
>
> I don't know?

Have you ever had a blood flow exam (Ankle Brachial Index - ABI)?

> Yes
>
> No
>
> I don't know?

Do you have calf or leg pain when walking that is improved with rest?

Yes

No

I don't know?

Step 3 - Skin and Wound Evaluation

Here are specific questions about the skin around your wound and the wound itself.

What is the size of your wound?

Measure it length, width and depth.

Can you see the bottom of your foot?

Using a mirror can help if you can't ask a family member or friend.

Yes

No

Do you have any redness, drainage or pain?

These are the signs of infection.If you have any of these, please visit your doctor.

Yes - you should see your doctor or emergency room

No

I don't know

Step 4 - Bone and Pressure Evaluation

Do you feel like there is a bone present under your wound?

Many times a bunion or prominent bone will not allow a foot wound to heal.

Yes

No

I don't know

Does your wound go down to the bone?

If you can feel or see bone though your ulcer it may be infected.

Yes

No

I don't know

Have you had an x-ray or MRI?

These tests can be done to determine if there is any bone infection in your foot under your foot wound.

Yes

No

Step 5 - Nerve and Feeling Evaluation

How is your feeling? If it is poor and you can't feel when walking on your foot, this could make your wound slow to heal.

Do you have numbness or tingling in your feet?

>Yes

>No

>I don't know

Have you been told you have neuropathy?

This would be determined by your doctor.

>Yes

>No

>I don't know

Does your wound hurt when you walk on it

If you can walk on your wound without pain that is a sign of lack of feeling or neuropathy.

>Yes

>No

>I don't know

Step 6 - Wound Debridement and Surgery

Is someone debriding (removing callus and tissue) from your wound on a regular basis?

>Yes

>No

>I don't know

Are you using and creams or wound coverings that use chemicals to debride your wound?

Yes

No

I don't know

Do you have a bone that needs to be removed or corrected to help heal your wound?

Hammertoes, Charcot foot and other prominences may need to be corrected to help your wound heal.

Yes

No

I don't know

Do you have a tight heel cord contributing to your foot wound?

Yes

No

I don't know

Step 7 - Wound Dressings and Grafts

Do you change your own foot dressings?

Yes

No

What type of dressing are you currently using on your wound?

No dressing I am not covering my wound

I am using only gauze

I am using betadine and gauze

I am using a hydrogel dressing (Amerigel)

I am using an alginate dressing (Aquacel AG)

I am using a collagen dressing (Promogran)

I don't know

Other:

Have you ever used a wound VAC?

A vacuum dressing to remove drainage on the wound

Yes

No

I don't know

Have you ever used a skin substitute?

Apligraf

Graftjacket

Dermagraft

I don't know

Other:

Do you have a nurse coming home to change your dressings?

Yes

No

Step 8 - Shoes and Off-loading

How are you keeping the pressure off your foot wound?

Write in your answer

Have you used a pedometer to see how much you are walking?

Yes

No

Are you using any of these off-loading shoes?

Surgical shoe

Off-loading boot with pegs

CROW walker

Ortho-Wedge Shoe

I don't know

Are you using any of these things?

Crutches

Wheelchair

Roll-About

Nothing

Step 9 - Preventing Recurrence and Other Complications

Do you look at your feet and your wound every day?

Yes

No

Do you see a podiatrist at least once a year?

Yes

No

Do you wear diabetic shoes?

Yes

No

CONCLUSION

I have tried to remove the technical words about wound healing and make the topic easy to understand. If you have any comments or suggestions please email me at don@centralmasspodiatry.com as this version at it will be updated in the future.

Please be advised this book is not to replace medical care and is only an educational resource if you have a foot wound or are treating foot wounds.

To your health,

Dr. Donald Pelto